Muscle-Building Cookbook

Lose Fat, Build Muscle

Over 25 Delicious Recipes to Help You Get the Body You Want

BY: Nancy Silverman

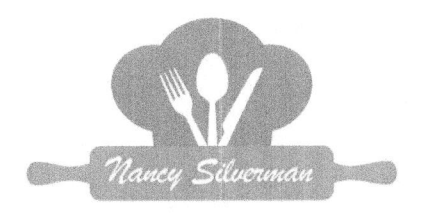

COPYRIGHT NOTICES

© **2019 Nancy Silverman All Rights Reserved**

Subject to the agreement and permission of the author, this Book, in part or in whole, may not be reproduced in any format. This includes but is not limited to electronically, in print, scanning or photocopying.

The opinions, guidelines and suggestions written here are solely those of the Author and are for information purposes only. Every possible measure has been taken by the Author to ensure accuracy but let the Reader be advised that they assume all risk when following information. The Author does not assume any risk in the case of damages, personally or commercially, in the case of misinterpretation or misunderstanding while following any part of the Book.

My Heartfelt Thanks and A Special Reward for Your Purchase!

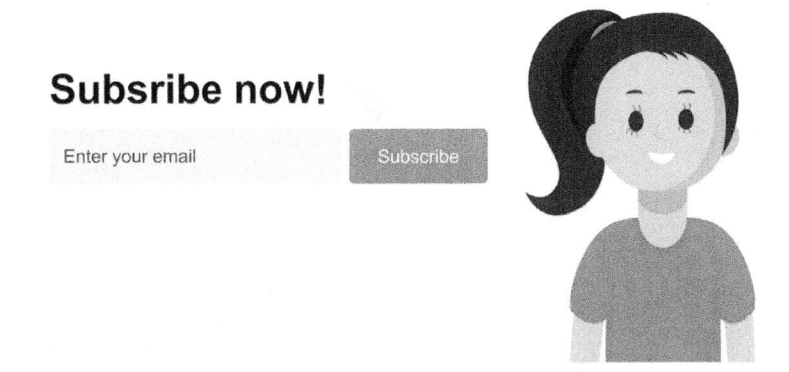

https://nancy.gr8.com

My heartfelt thanks at purchasing my book and I hope you enjoy it! As a special bonus, you will now be eligible to receive books absolutely free on a weekly basis! Get started by entering your email address in the box above to subscribe. A notification will be emailed to you of my free promotions, no purchase necessary! With little effort, you will be eligible for free and discounted books daily. In addition to this amazing gift, a reminder will be sent 1-2 days before the offer expires to remind you not to miss out. Enter now to start enjoying this special offer!

Table of Contents

Best Ways to Build Lean Muscle with Diet 7

    (1)   Take into Consideration How Much You Need to Eat 8

    (2)   What does this have to do with you? 9

    (3)   Take into Consideration How Much You Need to Eat 10

    (4)   What to Do Pre and Post Workout 11

Top 10 Muscle Friendly Foods to Consume 12

    (1)   Beef 13

    (2)   Eggs 14

    (3)   Salmon 15

    (4)   Rotisserie Chicken 16

    (5)   Nuts 17

    (6)   Protein Shakes 18

    (7)   Scallops 19

- (8) Cottage Cheese 20
- (9) Lentils 21
- (10) Chickpeas 22

Healthy Muscle Building Recipes 23

- (1) Protein Packed Snickerdoodle 24
- (2) Savory Cheeseburger Style Omelet 27
- (3) Breakfast Style Banana Split 29
- (4) Game Day Bulk Nachos 32
- (5) Protein Packed Chili Dogs 34
- (6) Crustless Pumpkin Pie 37
- (7) Delicious Chicken Burrito Bowl 39
- (8) Muscle Building Beef Enchiladas 42
- (9) Savory Strawberry Shortcake 45
- (10) Protein Packed White Chocolate Peppermint Bars ... 47
- (11) Low Carb Bacon and Ranch Potato Salad 49
- (12) Extra Lean Turkey Reuben 51

(13) Healthy Chicken and Waffles 53

(14) The Ultimate Muscle Mac 56

(15) Delicious Breakfast Burrito 59

(16) Sriracha Spiced Chicken and Cheese Fries 61

(17) Peanut Butter Chocolate Chip French Toast 63

(18) Low Carb Orange Chicken 65

(19) Decadent Protein Brownies 67

(20) Filling Sweet Potato Shepherd's Pie 70

(21) Delicious Cheesy Steak Pizza 72

(22) Decadent Chocolate and Banana Protein Bars 74

(23) Simple Tiramisu 76

(24) Protein Packed Ranch and Turkey Burger 78

(25) Protein Boosting Rice Pudding 80

About the Author 82

Author's Afterthoughts 84

Best Ways to Build Lean Muscle with Diet

When it comes to building lean muscle within your body, you need to think of your body as a machine that constantly needs to reinvent itself. You need to remember that every minute of every single day your body is breaking down its own tissues and replacing them with new stuff to make it stronger. This all comes down to the combination of foods that you eat and recycled material that your body uses from other tissues.

There are many different ways that you can build lean muscle in your body by utilizing a healthy muscle friendly diet. In this section you will learn about the many different ways that you can build lean muscle so that you can start getting ripped in the way that you want to sooner rather than later.

(1) Take into Consideration How Much You Need to Eat

A recent study conducted in 2007 from the Journal of Applied Physiology found that muscle size increases every day by at least .2%. This occurs during the first 20 days of strength training and has to be above the highest rate of muscle protein breakdown that usually occurs at the same time.

(2) What does this have to do with you?

This will help you understand that when it comes to building muscles that you will not get ripped immediately. When you are just starting out you may not notice much of a difference in muscle growth but after the first 20 days that's when you will start to see some progress. With this in mind the fastest way for you to grow and gain muscle is to make sure that you utilize as much protein as your body needs to build big muscles. You are going to have to take into consideration how much protein you need.

I highly recommend when going on a muscle friendly diet to consume at least .73 grams of protein for every pound of body weight per day. For example, if you are 180 pounds, you need to make sure that you get at least 130 grams of protein per day in order to see substantial muscle growth.

(3) Take into Consideration How Much You Need to Eat

Another part of building healthy muscle in your body is the act of protein synthesis. Protein synthesis is the simple process that takes the protein from the food that you eat and turns it into the muscle tissue within your body. This is very important because many of us tend to disregard the amount of protein that we take in daily.

In order to benefit from a diet that will help you build lean muscle, you need to ensure that you enjoy a low protein and high carb breakfast, a lunch that has a moderate amount of protein and a very high protein dinner.

Another thing that you need to keep in mind with protein synthesis is the fact that this usually peaks at around 16 hours after your main workout and it will remain elevated for the next 48 hours. So, what does this mean? Well this means that every meal that you have needs to count in order for you to build your lean and healthy muscle.

(4) What to Do Pre and Post Workout

In order to ensure that your protein synthesis peaks earlier and lasts much longer, you need to ensure that you pay attention to what you do pre and post-workout. A recent study conducted in 2012 from the American journal of Clinical Nutrition found that those who were taking protein supplements over the course of 12 weeks were able to gain at least two extra pounds in muscle opposed to those who didn't.

With that in mind it is always ideal for you to take a few protein supplements as well as enjoy a protein rich meal at least 2 or 3 hours before you actually train and at least one to two hours after you train.

Top 10 Muscle Friendly Foods to Consume

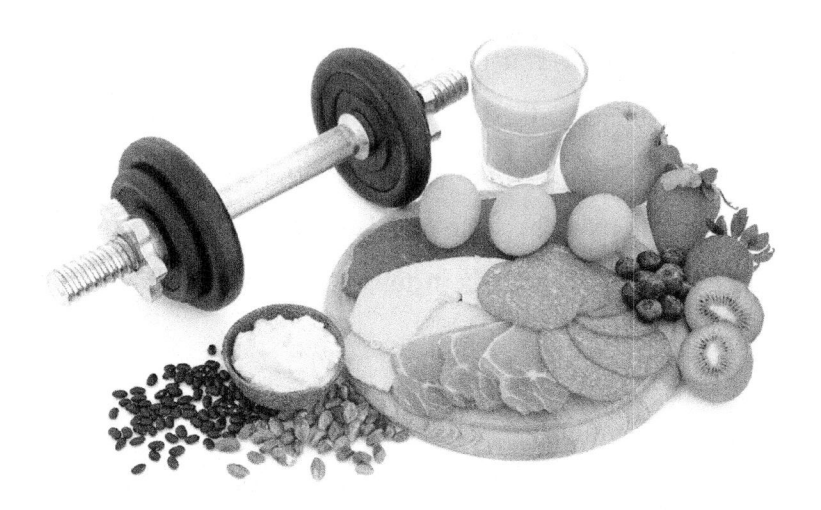

Now that you understand what it takes to build healthy lean muscle with in your body, it is time to actually see what types of foods you need to consume in order to build that muscle. In this section you will learn about the various different foods that you can enjoy helping build lean muscle while still filling yourself up and feeling satisfied as well.

(1) Beef

Beef is one of the best types of meat that you can consume if you want to build healthy and lean muscle. However, when it comes to beef, you need to make sure that you use extra lean beef so that you are not taking in too much fat in the process. Beef itself contains essential amino acids, various B vitamins and even creatine.

There are various benefits to consuming beef such as helping to support healthy testosterone levels, helping to promote healthy heart health and helping to reduce levels of anxiety and stress that a person may be suffering from.

(2) Eggs

Eggs themselves have been known to be a food that can potentially clog your arteries. However, further research has found that eggs have been able to help build serious muscle and it has been found that the link between cholesterol heart disease and eggs are almost non-existent. When it comes to muscle the cholesterol that is found in egg yolks serves as a scaffolding for the hormones that your body produces to build muscle. So, if you want to build lean muscle, make sure that you eat plenty of eggs.

(3) Salmon

Salmon is another high-quality source of protein that you are going to want to add to your diet on a daily basis. Salmon contains both omega 3 and 6 fatty acids which can help promote healthy hair and skin as well as help improve the health of your heart. This is a great high quality protein source to use as often as possible to help you build your lean muscles. If you are the type of person that does not like salmon, all that you have to do is make sure that you take a fish supplement instead.

(4) Rotisserie Chicken

There are going to be many times where you need to ensure that you get in some healthy muscle food as soon as possible. This is when rotisserie chicken can come into play as it can be used as your emergency muscle food. The best thing about rotisserie chicken is that you can easily find this in many local supermarkets, and it is ready to eat so that you can enjoy a protein in a delicious package.

(5) Nuts

Nuts are another great food to eat if you want to build lean and healthy muscle. Nuts contain the perfect combination of protein, fiber and fat which allows you to gain the extra calories without adding them to your waistline. Nuts are extremely easy to bring around with you so it is easy and convenient to snack on throughout the day if you need to increase the amount of calories you take in.

(6) Protein Shakes

When it comes to building healthy lean muscle, you need to make sure that you are taking in as much protein as possible. This is where protein and carbohydrate shake can be essential in your muscle building program. By consuming a shake that consist of protein and carbohydrates before your workout you can set the stage to build optimal muscle growth and ensure that you are getting all of the nutrients that you need.

This kind of shake can help increase blood flow to your muscles, improve your body's ability to process and use carbohydrates and even increase the regulation for creatine transport. All around this is incredibly healthy for you if you want to build muscle.

(7) Scallops

Similar to many different types of seafood, scallops are lean and rich in protein. They aren't only soft and tasty, but they contain as much as 15 grams of protein for every 3.5-ounce pack that you purchase. This is a great food product to pick up if you live near the coast or if you want to add a little extra flavor to your next muscle building meal.

(8) Cottage Cheese

Cottage cheese is another surprising muscle building food that you can consume whenever you wish. The way cottage cheese builds to build muscle comes from two different components such as it helps to fuel a high proportion of casein which helps your cells to digest protein found in dairy items as well as contain live bacteria that can help you break down and absorb all of the nutrients that your body needs in order to stay healthy and stronger in the long run.

(9) Lentils

If you are looking to build healthy muscles incredibly fast than lentils are something that you need to add into your everyday diet. It is the secret to building mass muscles as it contains almost 18 grams of protein with every cup. Lentils are also very inexpensive, making them convenient for those who do not want to use them all the time. They are easy to make and pair excellently with some brown rice, a healthy salad or can even be eaten by themselves.

(10) Chickpeas

Of course, you have already learned that legumes can be incredibly healthy for you as they are an excellent source of protein. Chickpeas themselves are a great source of carbohydrates as well and are considered to be one of the most versatile beans that you can enjoy. These beans contain at least 45 grams of carbs that are slow acting as well as contain up to 12 grams of fiber per cup. This is a great ingredient to use if you plan on getting big and staying lean for many years to come.

Healthy Muscle Building Recipes

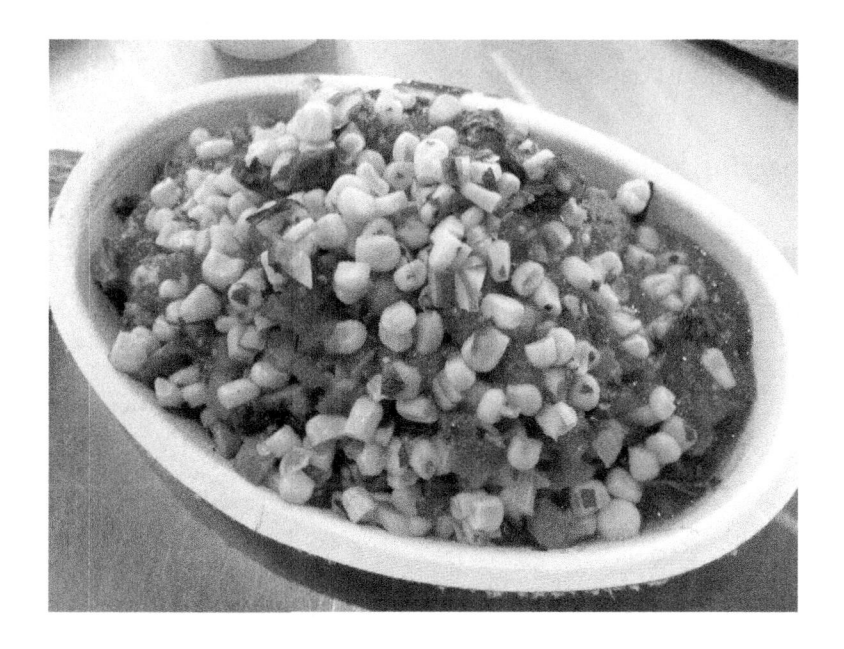

(1) Protein Packed Snickerdoodle

Here is yet another sweet tasting dessert dish that is packed with plenty of protein to help build your lean muscles. These make for the perfect holiday treat and I guarantee that even the pickiest eaters will love.

Serving Size: 1 Serving

Preparation Time: 40 Minutes

List of Ingredients:

- ¼ Cup of Flour, Coconut Variety
- 2 ½ Scoops of Protein Powder, Snickerdoodle Variety
- ¾ teaspoon of Baker's Style Baking Powder
- ½ teaspoon of Sea Salt, For Taste
- ¼ Cup of Honey, Raw
- 1 Egg, Large in Size
- 1 Tablespoon of Oil, Coconut Variety, Fully Melted
- 1 ½ teaspoon of Vanilla, Pure
- 2 teaspoon of Cinnamon, Ground
- 2 Tablespoon of Xylitol, Optional

Methods:

1. First sift together your coconut flour, baker's style baking powder, salt and protein powder until evenly mixed.

2. Then use a separate bowl and whisk together your melted coconut oil, beaten egg, vanilla and honey until evenly mixed.

3. Combine both your wet and dry ingredients until evenly mixed together. Cover with some plastic wrap and place into your fridge to chill for the next 20 minutes.

4. Meanwhile preheat your oven to 325 degrees. While your oven is heating up line a baking sheet with some parchment paper.

5. Use a small sized bowl and mix together your cinnamon and your Xylitol, if you wish.

6. After this time shape your dough into even sized balls and roll into your cinnamon mixture.

7. Place onto your baking sheet and flatten until it reaches your desired shape.

8. Place into your oven to bake for the next 10 minutes. After this time remove from your oven and allow to cool slightly before serving.

(2) Savory Cheeseburger Style Omelet

This is a great tasting breakfast recipe to put together if you are looking for the perfect dish to fill you up in the morning. Feel free to make this dish for breakfast, brunch or lunch. Regardless, I know you are going to love it.

Serving Size: 1 Serving

Preparation Time: 25 Minutes

List of Ingredients:

- 2 Eggs, Large in Size and Beaten
- ½ Cup of Egg Whites
- 4 Ounces of Beef, Lean and Ground
- ¼ Cup of Tomatoes, Fresh and Thinly Sliced
- 2 Tablespoon of Cheddar Cheese, Reduced Fat
- Some Pickles, For Topping and Optional
- Some Ketchup, For Topping and Optional
- Dash of Salt and Pepper, For Taste

Methods:

1. First whisk together your eggs and egg whites until thoroughly beaten.

2. Then heat up a large sized skillet placed over medium heat. Once your skillet is hot enough add in your eggs and cover with some aluminum foil. Cook until it reaches your desired doneness and remove from heat.

3. Using a separate skillet, cook up your ground beef with a seasoning of salt and pepper over medium heat until no longer pink. Once done place into your skillet with your eggs and push to the side.

4. Top off your ground beef with your tomatoes and pickles and fold over your eggs.

5. Sprinkle with some cheese and return to low heat. Cover with some aluminum foil and continue to cook until your cheese is slightly melted.

6. Remove from heat and serve with their ketchup and chives. Enjoy.

(3) Breakfast Style Banana Split

Do you remember when you weren't allowed to have dessert for dinner? Well, with this recipe you can enjoy this tasty treat early in the morning. It is packed full of delicious protein, making it perfect for you if you are looking to build some lean muscle.

Serving Size: 1 Serving

Preparation Time: 40 Minutes

List of Ingredients:

- 1 Banana, Small in Size
- 1 Cup of Yogurt, Non Fat Variety and Greek Variety
- 1/3 Scoop of Protein Powder, Chocolate Variety
- 1/3 Scoop of Protein Powder, Vanilla Variety
- 1/3 Scoop of Protein Powder, Strawberry Variety
- 2 Tablespoon of Strawberries, Finely Diced
- 2 Tablespoon of Pineapple, Finely Diced
- 1 Tablespoon of Chocolate Sauce, Sugar Free Variety
- 2 tablespoon of Whipped Topping, Fat Free Variety
- 1 Cherry, Maraschino Variety
- 1 Tablespoon of Walnuts, Finely Crushed
- Some Sweetener, Optional and as Desired

Methods:

1. The first thing that you want to do is evenly divided yogurt into three separate medium sized bowls.

2. Then mix your chocolate protein powder with one type of yogurt in one bowl while mixing your strawberry protein powder with your yogurt in the second bowl. Last mix your vanilla protein powder with your yogurt in your third bowl and make sure to stir all of them until thoroughly combined.

3. Place your bowls into your freezer to chill for the next 20 minutes.

4. While your yogurt is freezing, slice your banana in half lengthwise and place into a bowl.

5. After this time remove your yogurt and mix each bowl thoroughly.

6. Place each of your yogurts on top of your banana and finish off with your pineapples, strawberries, chocolate sauce, whipped topping, cherries, walnuts, and sweetener if you are using them. Serve right away and enjoy.

(4) Game Day Bulk Nachos

This is the perfect dish for you to make if you need a great tasting appetizer to serve up during the next football game. These nachos are not only incredibly delicious, but they are also packed with delicious protein that can help build lean muscle.

Serving Size: 1 Serving

Preparation Time: 20 Minutes

List of Ingredients:

- 4 Ounces of Tortilla Chips, Corn Variety
- 10 Ounces of Beef, Lean and Ground
- 2 to 3 Tablespoon of Taco Seasoning, Low in Sodium
- 1 Cup of Tomatoes, Fresh and Thinly Sliced
- 1/3 Cup of Yogurt, Plain and Greek Variety
- ¼ Cup of Cheese, Cheddar Variety and Reduced in Fat
- ½ of a Medium Avocado, Finely Diced
- ½ Cup of Black Beans, Drained and Rinsed

Methods:

1. The first thing that you will want to do is cook your meat in a large sized skillet placed over medium heat until fully cooked through.

2. Once cooked through add in your taco seasoning and stir to thoroughly combine.

3. Place your tortilla chips onto a large sized serving plate.

4. Top off your chips with some cooked ground beef, cheese, tomato, black beans and avocado.

5. Finish off with a dollop of your yogurt. Serve right away and enjoy.

(5) Protein Packed Chili Dogs

If you are looking for a great way to use your grill, this is the perfect dish for you. These chili dogs are a great way to satisfy your taste buds and help you gain muscle at the same time.

Serving Size: 3 Servings

Preparation Time: 10 Minutes

Ingredients for Your Chili:

- 1 Pound of Turkey Breast, Lean and Ground
- 8 Ounces of Tomato Sauce, No Sodium Added
- 2 teaspoon of Chili
- 1 teaspoon of Garlic, Powdered Variety
- 1 teaspoon of Cumin, Ground
- 1 teaspoon of Black Pepper, For Taste
- 1 teaspoon of Red Pepper, Crushed Variety
- ½ teaspoon of Salt, For Taste
- Dash of Cinnamon, Ground and Optional

Ingredients for Your Hotdogs:

- 6 Hot Dogs, Low Fat Variety and Turkey Variety
- 6 Hot Dog Rolls, Light Variety
- Some Mustard, For Topping and Optional
- Some Cheese, For Topping and Optional
- Some Homemade Coleslaw, For Topping and Optional

Methods:

1. First use a large sized bowl and mix together your turkey breast, tomato sauce, powdered chili, garlic, cumin, dash of pepper and salt, crushed red pepper and ground cinnamon until thoroughly combined.

2. Place this mixture into a pan set over medium to high heat and cook for the next 3 to 4 minutes, making sure to stir thoroughly as it cooks.

3. Then reduce the heat to low and allow to simmer for the next five minutes.

4. After this time place your hot dogs onto a grill and cook until your hot dogs are done to your desired likeness. Once done cooking, place onto a hot dog bun and top off with your homemade chili. Top off with your onions and enjoy right away.

(6) Crustless Pumpkin Pie

If you are a huge fan of traditional pumpkin pie, then this is the perfect dish for you. It is packed full of delicious protein and makes for a delicious way to finish off your Thanksgiving or Christmas dinner.

Serving Size: 1 Serving

Preparation Time: 7 Hour

List of Ingredients:

- 2 Eggs, Large in Size and Beaten
- 1 ½ Cup of Yogurt, Non Fat Variety, Plain and Greek Variety
- 1, 15 Ounce Can of Pumpkin, Pure Variety
- 4 Scoops of Protein Powder, Whey Variety and Snickerdoodle Flavored
- 2 Tablespoon of Pumpkin Pie Spice
- Some Sweetened, Optional
- Whipped Topping, Topping and Optional
- Some Maple Syrup, Topping and Optional

Methods:

1. Preheat your oven to 325 degrees. While your oven is heating up spray a pie dish with some nonstick cooking spray and set aside for later use.

2. Place all of your ingredients into a large sized bowl and mix thoroughly until evenly combined.

3. Pour your mixture into your greased pie dish.

4. Place into your oven to bake for the next 45 to 50 minutes or until your pie is fully set.

5. Remove from your oven and allow to cool slightly before placing into your fridge to chill for next four to six hours.

6. After this time top your pie with some maple syrup or whipped cream. Serve right away and enjoy.

(7) Delicious Chicken Burrito Bowl

If you love Chipotle burrito bowls, then this is the perfect recipe for you. Mixed together with the perfect combination cilantro lime rice, guacamole and chicken, this is one dish that is you won't be able to get enough of.

Serving Size: 2 Servings

Preparation Time: 30 Minutes

List of Ingredients:

- 2 Cups of White Rice, Cooked
- 1 Lime, For Fresh
- 2 Tablespoon of Cilantro, Fresh and Roughly Chopped
- 12 Ounces of Chicken Breasts, Raw

Ingredients for Your Mexican Seasoning:

- 1/3 Cup of Black Beans, No Sodium Added
- ½ Cup of Pico de Gallo, Fresh
- ¼ Cup of Guacamole
- ¼ Cup of Yogurt, Non Fat Variety and Greek Variety
- ¼ Cup of Cheddar Cheese, Finely Shredded
- 1 Cup of Lettuce, Fresh and Finely Shredded

Methods:

1. The first thing that you want to do is toss your white rice with your lime and cilantro. Season with a dash of salt.

2. Season your chicken with your Mexican seasoning and place onto a preheated grill. Cook until it reaches your desired likeness. Once done chop up into small sized pieces.

3. Then warm up your black beans in your microwave.

4. Next use two decent sized serving bowls and divide up your cilantro lime rice, shredded lettuce, chicken breast, black beans, guacamole, pico de gallo and Greek yogurt evenly between both of them.

5. The top each bowl off with some cheddar cheese and a lime wedge. Serve whenever you are ready.

(8) Muscle Building Beef Enchiladas

Here is yet another Mexican inspired dish that I know you are going to fall in love with. Not only is this a great way to satisfy your cravings as well as an excellent way to build healthy and huge muscles.

Serving Size: 1 Serving

Preparation Time: 15 Minutes

List of Ingredients:

- 3 Tortillas, Low Carb Variety and High Protein Variety
- 4 Ounces of Beef, Ground and Lean
- ¼ Cup of Black Beans, No Salt, Drained and Rinsed
- ¼ Cup of Enchilada Sauce, Green or Red
- 2 Tablespoon of Green Chiles, Finely Diced
- ¼ Cup of Mexican Cheese, Low in Fat
- Dash of Salt and Pepper, For Taste
- Dash of Green Onions, If Desired

Methods:

1. The first thing you want to do is preheat your oven to 350 degrees.

2. While your oven is heating up use a large sized skillet placed over medium heat and cook up your ground beef until thoroughly cooked through.

3. Then add in your chilies along with a dash of salt and pepper and stir thoroughly to combine.

4. Transfer your meat to a separate medium sized bowl and add in your beans. Stir again to combine.

5. Spread at least half of your enchilada sauce into the bottom of a large sized baking dish.

6. Spread your meat and beans evenly between 3 tortillas and sprinkle with half of your cheese. Roll up your tortillas tightly and place the seam side down into your baking dish.

7. Spread your remaining enchilada sauce over the top and top off with some more shredded cheese.

8. Place into your oven to bake for the next 10 to 12 minutes.

9. After this time remove and allow to cool slightly before serving with your green onions, diced avocado and your yogurt. Enjoy.

(9) Savory Strawberry Shortcake

What is better than strawberry shortcake? If this is one of your favorite dishes, then I know you are going to want to make this dish over and over again. This is a healthy variation of strawberry shortcake that will help you build lean muscle.

Serving Size: 4 Servings

Preparation Time: 15 Minutes

List of Ingredients:

- ¾ Cup of Flour, Oat Variety
- 2 Scoops of Protein Powder, Vanilla Variety
- ½ Cup of Egg Whites, Vanilla Variety
- ½ teaspoon of Baker's Style Baking Soda
- Some Sweetened, As Desired
- 1 Cup of Yogurt, Greek Variety and Nonfat Variety
- 1 Cup of Strawberries, Fresh and Finely Diced

Methods:

1. The first thing that you want to do is preheat your grill to 350 degrees. While your oven is heating up spray a large sized muffin pan with some cooking spray and set aside for later use.

2. Then use a large sized bowl and whisk together your oat flour, protein powder and baker's style baking soda until thoroughly mixed together.

3. Then add in your egg whites and sweetener and stir thoroughly to combine. Allow your batter to sit for the next 5 minutes before pouring into your muffin pan.

4. Place into your oven to bake for the next 7 minutes. After this time remove from your oven and allow to cool for the next five minutes.

5. Once cooled cut out a small section of your muffin right in the center to make a cup and fill each center with your Greek yogurt. Top off with your strawberries and whipped cream and serve right away.

(10) Protein Packed White Chocolate Peppermint Bars

This is the perfect dish to serve up during the holiday season as well as whenever you wish to satisfy your strongest sweet tooth. Best of all you don't need to worry about baking this bars.

Serving Size: 1 Serving

Preparation Time: 1 Day

List of Ingredients:

- 1 Cup of Peanut Butter, White Chocolate Variety
- 5 Scoops of Protein Powder, White Chocolate Variety
- ¼ Cup of Flour, Coconut Variety
- ¼ Cup of Honey, Raw
- ¼ Cup of Oil, Coconut Variety
- ¼ Cup of Peppermint Candies, Crushed
- Some Milk, if Needed

Methods:

1. First sift together your coconut flour and protein powder until evenly mixed together.

2. Then use a separate bowl and melt your coconut oil until fully melted. Add in your peanut butter and sweetener and mix until thoroughly combined.

3. Add your dry ingredients to your wet ingredients and mix well to combine.

4. Next line a baking dish with some parchment paper and spread your mixture evenly onto your pan.

5. Top with your crushed peppermint and press lightly into your bars.

6. Set into your fridge to chill overnight or until completely set.

7. The next day cut up your bars into desired pieces and serve whenever you are ready.

(11) Low Carb Bacon and Ranch Potato Salad

This is the perfect dish to serve up for your next summer barbecue. Feel free to serve up this healthy side dish to accompany any entrée that you make.

Serving Size: 2 Servings

Preparation Time: 10 Minutes

List of Ingredients:

- 6 Cups of Cauliflower, Florets Only
- ½ Cup of Yogurt, Nonfat and Greek Variety
- 2 Tablespoon of Ranch Seasoning
- Dash of Salt and Pepper, For Taste
- ¼ Cup of Cheddar Cheese, Finely Shredded
- 1 to 2 Slices of Bacon, Cooked and Crumbled

Methods:

1. The first thing that you want to do is add your cauliflower to a large sized pot set over medium heat. Cover with some water and bring this mixture to a boil for the next 7 to 8 minutes or until tender to the touch. After this time drain your cauliflower and set aside for later use.

2. Next use a medium sized bowl and combine your Greek yogurt, dash of salt and pepper and ranch seasoning until thoroughly mixed together. Gently pour this over your cauliflower and mix until well coated.

3. Add in your cheddar cheese and crumbled bacon and continue to mix until thoroughly combined.

4. Serve with a garnish of chives and enjoy.

(12) Extra Lean Turkey Reuben

With this delicious dish you are able to bring the best of New York City into your household. This is a sandwich that is high in protein and low in fat, making it the most delicious sandwich to eat to gain muscle.

Serving Size: 1 Serving

Preparation Time: 10 Minutes

List of Ingredients:

- 2 Slices of Rye Bread, Light
- 5 Ounces of Turkey Breast, Thinly Sliced and Deli Variety
- 1 Slice of Swiss Cheese, Low in Fat
- 2 Tablespoon of Sauerkraut
- ½ Tablespoon of Thousand Island Dressing, Light Variety
- Dash of Salt and Pepper, For Taste

Methods:

1. The first thing that you will want to do his toast your bread until it reaches your desired doneness.

2. Then layer one slice of your toasted bread with your turkey breast, sauerkraut and cheese. Drizzle your dressing over the top and top off with your second piece of toast.

3. Slice your sandwich in half and serve with a deli pickle for an authentic New York City experience.

(13) Healthy Chicken and Waffles

While I know this dish may not seem like a great tasting combination, but once you get a taste of it I know you will think differently. Feel free to top this dish off with some soul food to make it incredibly delicious.

Serving Size: 2 Servings

Preparation Time: 45 Minutes

List of Ingredients:

- 1 Cup of Pancake Mix, Protein Variety
- 12 Ounces of Chicken Breasts, Boneless and Skinless Variety
- ½ Cup of Milk, Low Fat Variety
- 1 to 2 Tablespoon of Hot Sauce, Your Favorite Kind
- 1 Cup of Special K, High Protein
- 4 ½ Tablespoon of Cornmeal, Yellow Variety
- 1 Tablespoon of Paprika
- Dash of Salt and Pepper, For Taste
- Some Syrup, For Topping and Optional
- Some Powdered Sugar, For Topping and Optional

Methods:

1. The first thing that you want to do is add your milk, hot sauce and chicken into a large sized Ziploc bag and shake thoroughly coat your chicken. Then place your chicken in your fridge to sit overnight.

2. The next day place your special K cereal into a food processor and blend on the highest setting until coarse in consistency. Then add to another large sized Ziploc bag along with your cornmeal, paprika and dash of salt and pepper.

3. Preheat your oven to 400 Degrees. While your oven is heating up line a baking sheet with some parchment paper and set aside for later use.

4. Then remove your chicken one piece at a time and place into your cereal mixture. Shake thoroughly until coated and repeat until all of your chicken is coated.

5. Place your coated chicken onto your baking sheet and place into your oven to bake for the next 20 minutes.

6. After this time reduce the heat of your oven to 350 degrees and bake for an additional 15 minutes or until crispy to the touch.

7. While your chicken is cooking make your waffles according to the directions on the package and place onto serving plates.

8. Top your waffles with your cooked chicken and serve with some butter and syrup if desired.

(14) The Ultimate Muscle Mac

If you are looking for the ultimate way to boost your muscle mass while enjoying a delicious meal, this is the perfect dish for you. This burger is delicious and great for you to build healthy and lean muscle in no time.

Serving Size: 1 Serving

Preparation Time: 15 Minutes

List of Ingredients:

- 1 ½ Sesame Buns, Your Favorite Kind
- 2 to 4 Ounces of Beef Patties, Ground and Lean
- 2 Leaves of Lettuce, Fresh
- 4 Pickle Slices, Fresh
- 1 Slice of Cheddar Cheese, Reduced in Fat

Ingredients for Your Special Sauce:

- ¼ Cup of Yogurt, Nonfat and Greek Variety
- ½ Tablespoon of Ketchup, Your Favorite Kind
- Dash of Garlic, Powdered Variety
- Dash of Onion, Powdered Variety
- Dash of Black Pepper and Salt, For Taste
- 2 Tablespoon of Protein Powder, Unflavored and Optional

Methods:

1. The first thing that you will want to do is mix together all of your ingredients for your sauce until thoroughly mixed together.

2. Next grill your hamburgers as you desire and spread at least half of your special sauce onto the bottom of your hamburger buns.

3. Top off with your lettuce and a hamburger patty before topping off with your bottom bun. Then add your special sauce over the top of this bun as well as your lettuce, pickles and second hamburger patty.

4. Place your top bun on top and serve right away.

(15) Delicious Breakfast Burrito

This is the perfect dish to make if you are looking for a meal to take along with you when you need to rush to work. Best of all, this is a dish that you can make if you are ever craving Mexican cuisine.

Serving Size: 2 Servings

Preparation Time: 30 Minutes

List of Ingredients:

- 4 Tortillas, Low Carb Variety
- 2 Eggs, Large in Size
- 1 Cup of Egg Whites, Beaten Lightly
- 4 Ounces of Beef, Lean and Ground
- ½ Cup of Cheddar Cheese, Finely Shredded and Low in Fat
- ½ of a Green Pepper, Finely Diced
- ½ of a Red Pepper, Finely Diced
- ½ of an Onion, Small in Size and Finely Diced
- 1 ½ Tablespoon of Taco Seasoning
- Dash of Pepper and Salt, For Taste

Methods:

1. First use a medium sized bowl and whisk together your eggs and your egg whites until thoroughly beaten.

2. Next spray a medium sized skillet with some nonstick cooking spray and cook your eggs with some salt and pepper if you want over medium heat until it reaches your desired doneness. Once fully cooked remove from pan and cover for later use.

3. Next add in your ground beef and taco seasoning to your skillet and cook until your beef is no longer pink. This should take about 5 to 10 minutes.

4. Place your tortilla onto a plate and layer your scrambled eggs, peppers, onions, cooked ground beef and cheese over the tortilla.

5. Wrap up burrito style and serve with a side of fresh fruit for the tastiest results. Enjoy.

(16) Sriracha Spiced Chicken and Cheese Fries

If you are looking for a way to spice up your dinner, this is the perfect dish for you. It is definitely the perfect way to add a bit of heat to your day.

Serving Size: 1 Serving

Preparation Time: 35 Minutes

List of Ingredients:

- 4 Sweet Potatoes, Medium in Size, White in Color and Sliced Thinly
- 1 Cup of Cheddar Cheese, Reduced Fat
- 1 ½ Cup of Chicken Breasts, Raw
- ¼ Cup of Sriracha Sauce, Your Favorite Kind
- Some Chives, For Topping and Optional

Methods:

1. The first thing that you want to do is preheat your oven to 425 degrees. While your oven is heating up coat a large sized baking dish with some cooking spray and set aside for later use.

2. Add in your potatoes/fries into your baking dish and place into your preheated oven to bake for the next 20 minutes.

3. While your potatoes are baking, boil your chicken in a pot filled with water until fully cook through. After this time shred up your chicken using two forks and toss with your Sriracha sauce.

4. Remove your fries from your oven and top with your shredded chicken and cheese.

5. Place back into your oven to bake for the next 6 to 7 minutes. After this time remove and top off with your chives before serving. Enjoy.

(17) Peanut Butter Chocolate Chip French Toast

This is the perfect way to start off your day every morning. Packed with plenty of protein to help you build lean muscle, I know this is one dish that you will want to serve up over and over again.

Serving Size: 1 Serving

Preparation Time: 15 Minutes

List of Ingredients:

- 4 Slices of Whole Wheat Bread, Whole and Thinly Sliced
- ½ Scoop of Protein Powder, Vanilla Variety
- 1 Tablespoon of Sweetener, Granulated Variety
- ½ teaspoon of Cinnamon, Ground
- 2 Eggs, Whole and Large in Size
- ½ Cup of Milk, Whole
- 2 Tablespoon of Peanut Butter, Smooth Variety
- 1 teaspoon of Chocolate Chips, Mini Variety
- 2 Chocolate Chip Cookies, Optional and Mini

Methods:

1. The first thing that you want to do is preheat a griddle to medium or high heat.

2. While your grill is heating up whisk together your egg, ground cinnamon, whole milk and protein powder until thoroughly mixed.

3. Soak each slice of bread in your egg mixture on both sides. Place onto your griddle to cook for the next 3 minutes or until golden brown in color. Flip and cook until golden. This should take at least 3 minutes as well.

4. Next heat up your peanut butter until fully melted. Drizzle all over your French toast and top off with your chocolate chips.

5. Serve right away and enjoy.

(18) Low Carb Orange Chicken

Here is a dish that will help you keep your carbs low and your protein levels high, making this a muscle builders dream. It is incredibly delicious and packed full of tangy flavor that you won't be able to resist.

Serving Size: 1 Serving

Preparation Time: 45 Minutes

List of Ingredients:

- 1 Pound of Chicken Breast, Raw
- 6 Tablespoon of Marmalade, Orange Variety
- 1 Tablespoon of Soy Sauce, Your Favorite Kind
- ½ teaspoon of Vinegar, Apple Cider Variety
- Dash of Garlic, Powdered Variety
- Dash of Onion, Powdered Variety
- Dash of Sesame Seeds, Optional

Methods:

1. First cut your chicken into bite sized pieces.

2. Then heat up a large sized skillet placed over medium heat. Once your skillet is hot enough add in your chicken breast and cook for the next 2 minutes.

3. Then add in your onion and garlic powder and stir to combine. Continue cooking for the next five minutes.

4. While your chicken is cooking mix together your orange marmalade, favorite soy sauce and vinegar until thoroughly combined. Add in a bit of honey if you wish to have your sauce sweet to taste.

5. Once your chicken is fully cooked reduce the heat to low and add in your sauce. Toss thoroughly to coat.

6. Cover and continue cooking until your sauce is thick in consistency.

7. Remove from heat and garnish with your sesame seeds before serving.

(19) Decadent Protein Brownies

Want to enjoy delicious brownies in an incredibly healthy way? Then you can't go wrong with this recipe. With this recipe you can easily indulge yourself while your muscles thank you in the process.

Serving Size: 8 Servings

Preparation Time: 40 Minutes

List of Ingredients:

- ½ Cup of Milk, Almond Variety
- ½ Cup of Egg Whites, Chocolate Variety
- ¼ Cup of Apple Sauce
- ½ Cup + 1 Tablespoon of Yogurt, Non Fat and Greek Variety
- 1 Cup of Flour, Oat Variety
- 2 Scoops of Protein Powder, Chocolate Variety
- 3 Tablespoon of Cocoa Powder, Unsweetened Variety
- 1 teaspoon of Baker's Style Baking Soda
- ½ teaspoon of Salt, For Taste

Ingredients for Your Frosting:

- ½ Cup of Yogurt, Non Fat and Greek Variety
- ¼ Cup of Cherries, Fresh
- Some Sweetened, Optional and as Desired

IIIIIIIIIIIIIIIIIIIIIIIIIIIIIIIIIIIIIIIIIIIIIIIIII

Methods:

1. The first thing that you want to do is preheat your oven to 350 degrees. While your oven is heating up spray a large sized baking dish with some non-stick cooking spray and set aside for later use.

2. Then mix together your whole milk, egg whites, Greek yogurt and applesauce in a medium sized bowl until evenly mixed.

3. Then use a second bowl and whisk together your oat flour, sweetener, baker's style baking soda, powdered cocoa and protein powder until evenly mixed.

4. Add your dry ingredients to your wet mixture and continue to stir until evenly combined. Allow your batter to sit for the next five minutes.

5. Pour your batter into your baking dish and place into your oven to bake for the next 20 to 25 minutes or until completely baked through.

6. While your brownies are cooking place your cherries, sweetener and Greek yogurt into a food processor and blend until smooth in consistency.

7. Remove your brownies from your oven and allow to cool slightly. Serve with your yogurt mixture and enjoy whenever you are ready.

(20) Filling Sweet Potato Shepherd's Pie

This is a dish that you will want to make if you are looking for the ultimate comfort food. It is a great way to ensure you get your daily dose of protein without straying away from your diet in the process.

Serving Size: 1 Serving

Preparation Time: 1 Hour and 10 Minutes

List of Ingredients:

- 2 Pounds of Beef, Lean and Ground
- 6 Ounces of Tomato Paste, No Salt Variety
- 1 to 12 Ounces of Veggies, Frozen and Your Favorite Kind
- Dash of Garlic, Powdered Variety
- Dash of Onion, Powdered Variety
- Dash of Salt and Pepper, For Taste
- 2 ½ Cups of Sweet Potatoes, Mashed
- Dash of Paprika

Methods:

1. First preheat your oven to 375 degrees.

2. While your oven is heating up add in your ground beef to a large sized skillet and cook over medium heat until no longer pink.

3. Once your beef has been fully cooked add in your tomato paste, frozen veggies and seasonings. Stir thoroughly to combine and continue to cook the next 5 minutes or until your veggies are soft to the touch.

4. Then add in your mixture to a large sized baking dish and spread your mashed sweet potatoes over the top of it.

5. Sprinkle a dash of paprika over the top and place into your oven to bake for the next 35 to 40 minutes.

6. After this time remove from the oven and allow to cool slightly before serving.

(21) Delicious Cheesy Steak Pizza

Forget delivery! With this delicious recipe now you can enjoy a mouthwatering pizza without having to spend the extra buck. It is incredibly easy to prepare and can help boost the amount of protein you take in per day.

Serving Size: 3 Servings

Preparation Time: 40 Minutes

List of Ingredients:

- 1, 12 Inch Pizza Crust, Premade and Your Favorite Kind
- 1 Cup of Pizza Sauce
- 1 Cup of Mozzarella Cheese, reduced in Fat and Finely Shredded
- ½ Cup of Green Peppers, Thinly Sliced
- ½ of an Onion, Red in Color and Thinly Sliced
- 12 Ounces of Steak, Lean and Raw

Methods:

1. The first thing that you want to do is slice your steak into thin sized strips and place into a pan placed over medium to high heat. Cook until it reaches your desired doneness and remove from heat to set aside for later use.

2. Next preheat your oven to 375 degrees. While your oven is heating up, line a baking sheet with parchment paper and set aside for later use.

3. Place your pizza crust onto your baking sheet and top off with half of your cheese, peppers, onions and freshly grilled steak. Top off with your remaining cheese.

4. Place into your oven for the next 40 minutes or until golden in color and the cheese is bubbly.

5. Remove from your oven and allow to cool slightly before serving.

(22) Decadent Chocolate and Banana Protein Bars

If you are looking for a cheap way to help satisfy your sweet teeth and build healthy muscle at the same time, then this is the recipe for you. These bars are inexpensive and big on flavor. You will fall in love with these!

Serving Size: 1 Serving

Preparation Time: 15 Minutes

List of Ingredients:

- 4 ½ Scoops of Protein Powder, Banana Cream Variety
- 1/3 Cup of Flour, Coconut Variety
- 1/3 Cup of Milk, Almond Variety
- 2 Tablespoon of Chocolate Chips, Miniature Variety
- 1/8 teaspoon of Stevia, Liquid Variety
- ¼ teaspoon of Vanilla, Pure

Methods:

1. First sift together your coconut flour and protein powder until evenly mixed.

2. Place into a large sized bowl and add in your vanilla, almond milk and stevia. Mix thoroughly for the next 5 minutes until combined.

3. Once your dough has been formed, mix in your chocolate chips and gently stir.

4. Evenly divide up your dough and shape it into even sized bars. Place into your freezer to chill until you are ready to eat them.

(23) Simple Tiramisu

Here is yet another decadent dessert dish that I know you are going to love. It is a great way to satisfy your sweet tooth while helping you to gain muscle in the process.

Serving Size: 4 Servings

Preparation Time: 1 Day and 20 Minutes

List of Ingredients:

- 1 Box of Lady Fingers
- 3 Cups of Yogurt, Non Fat Variety and Greek Style
- 1 ½ Cups of Whey Protein Powder, Vanilla Flavored
- 1 ½ teaspoon of Vanilla
- 4 to 5 Drops of Stevia, Liquid Variety and Optional
- 2 teaspoons of Cinnamon, Ground
- 2 teaspoons of Cocoa
- 1 Cup of Coffee, Strong
- 1 Piece of Chocolate, Dark and Sugar Free

Methods:

1. Use a large sized bowl and combine your Greek yogurt, protein powder, Stevia and vanilla until thoroughly mixed. Then use an electric mixer and beat for the next 45 to 60 seconds or until everything is fully combined.

2. Soak your lady fingers one at a time in your coffee mixture and place into the bottom of a large sized generously greased baking dish. Place a layer of cookies over the top.

3. Top off your cookies with at least one third of your yogurt mixture, ground cinnamon and powdered cocoa. Repeat your layers until all of your ingredients have been used.

4. Place into your fridge to sit overnight until fully set.

5. The next day serve your dish with a dollop of your favorite whipped cream and serve whenever you are ready.

(24) Protein Packed Ranch and Turkey Burger

If you are looking for the ultimate filling burger to enjoy for lunch or for dinner, this is the perfect dish for you. For the tastiest results feel free to use whatever toppings you desire.

Serving Size: 1 Serving

Preparation Time: 5 Minutes

List of Ingredients:

- 1 Hamburger Roll, Whole Wheat Variety
- 6 Ounces of Turkey Breast
- 1 teaspoon of Ranch Seasoning
- Lettuce, Fresh and for Topping
- Some Tomato, Thinly Sliced and for Topping
- Some Condiments, For Topping

Methods:

1. Mix together your turkey breast and ranch seasoning until thoroughly mixed.

2. Preheat a grill to medium or high heat and once it is hot enough grill your turkey burgers until they reach your desired doneness.

3. Remove from your grill and place onto a hamburger roll.

4. Serve with your lettuce and tomatoes and enjoy right away.

(25) Protein Boosting Rice Pudding

If you are a huge fan of rice pudding, then I know this is the perfect dish for you. It is incredibly delicious and one of the sweetest way to add some lean muscles to your body. I know you won't regret making this dish.

Serving Size: 4 Servings

Preparation Time: 30 Minutes

List of Ingredients:

- 2 Cups of Brown Rice, Fully Cooked
- 2 Cups of Almond Milk, Unsweetened Variety
- ½ Cup of Protein Powder, Cinnamon Variety
- 2 Tablespoon of Butter, Reduced Fat
- 1 teaspoon of Cinnamon, Ground Variety
- 1 teaspoon of Vanilla, Pure
- Some Stevia, Optional
- Some Raisins, Optional
- Whipped Topping, Optional

Methods:

1. The first thing that you will want to do is combine your cooked rice, almond milk, soft butter, ground cinnamon and vanilla in a medium sized pot set over medium heat.

2. Bring your mixture to a simmer and reduce the heat to low. Continue to cook for the next 7 to 10 minutes or until your mixture begins to thicken in consistency. Make sure that you stir continuously as it does so.

3. Then add in your protein powder and remaining milk and continue to cook for the next 10 to 12 minutes or until thick and creamy in consistency.

4. Turn off the heat and allow your mixture to cook for the next to the 3 minutes before removing completely from heat. Allow to cool for at least 20 minutes.

5. After this time place in your fridge for the next 3 to 4 hours to cool completely.

6. After this time serve with your raisins garnished over the top and enjoy.

About the Author

Nancy Silverman is an accomplished chef and cookbook author from Essex, Vermont. She attended Essex High School where she graduated with honors then moved on to University of Vermont where she received a degree in Nutrition and Food Sciences. She later attended New England Culinary Institute located close to her home town of Essex, in Montpelier, Vermont.

Nancy met her husband at school in Vermont when the two were set up on a date by a mutual friend. Both shared a love of the culinary arts and it was love at first sight! Nancy and Dennis have been married for 16 years and live on a beautiful property close to Nancy's childhood home in Essex. They have 3 children and 2 golden retrievers named Lucy and Ricky.

Nancy loves growing her own vegetables and herbs in the garden she has cultivated and cared for in the family's spacious backyard. Her greatest joy is cooking in her modern kitchen with her family and creating inspiring and delicious meals. She often says that she has perfected her signature dishes based on her family's critique of each and every one.

Nancy has her own catering company and has also been fortunate enough to be head chef at some of Vermont's most exclusive restaurants. She aspires to open her own restaurant, but for now she is content working from home and building her catering empire with the help of her children. When a friend suggested she share some of her outstanding signature dishes, she decided to add cookbook author to her repertoire of personal achievements. Being a technological savvy woman, she felt the e-book realm would be a better fit and soon she had her first cookbook available online. As of today, Nancy has sold over 1,000 e-books and has shared her culinary experiences and brilliant recipes with people from all over the world! She plans on expanding into self-help books and dietary cookbooks, so stayed tuned!

Author's Afterthoughts

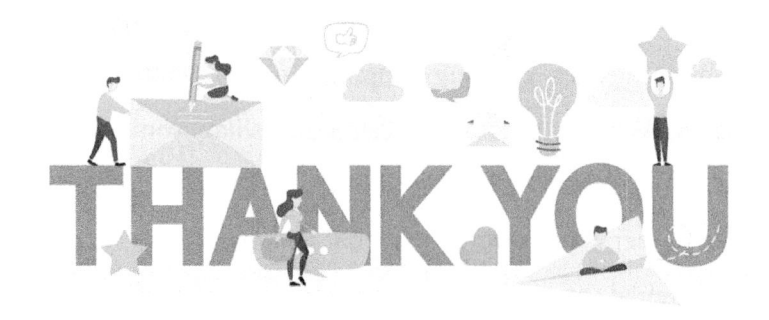

Thank you for making the decision to invest in one of my cookbooks! I cherish all my readers and hope you find joy in preparing these meals as I have.

There are so many books available and I am truly grateful that you decided to buy this one and follow it from beginning to end.

I love hearing from my readers on what they thought of this book and any value they received from reading it. As a personal favor, I would appreciate any feedback you can give in the form of a review on Amazon and please be honest! This kind of support will help others make an informed choice on and will help me tremendously in producing the best quality books possible.

My most heartfelt thanks,

Nancy Silverman

If you're interested in more of my books, be sure to follow my author page on Amazon (can be found on the link Bellow) or scan the QR-Code.

https://www.amazon.com/author/nancy-silverman

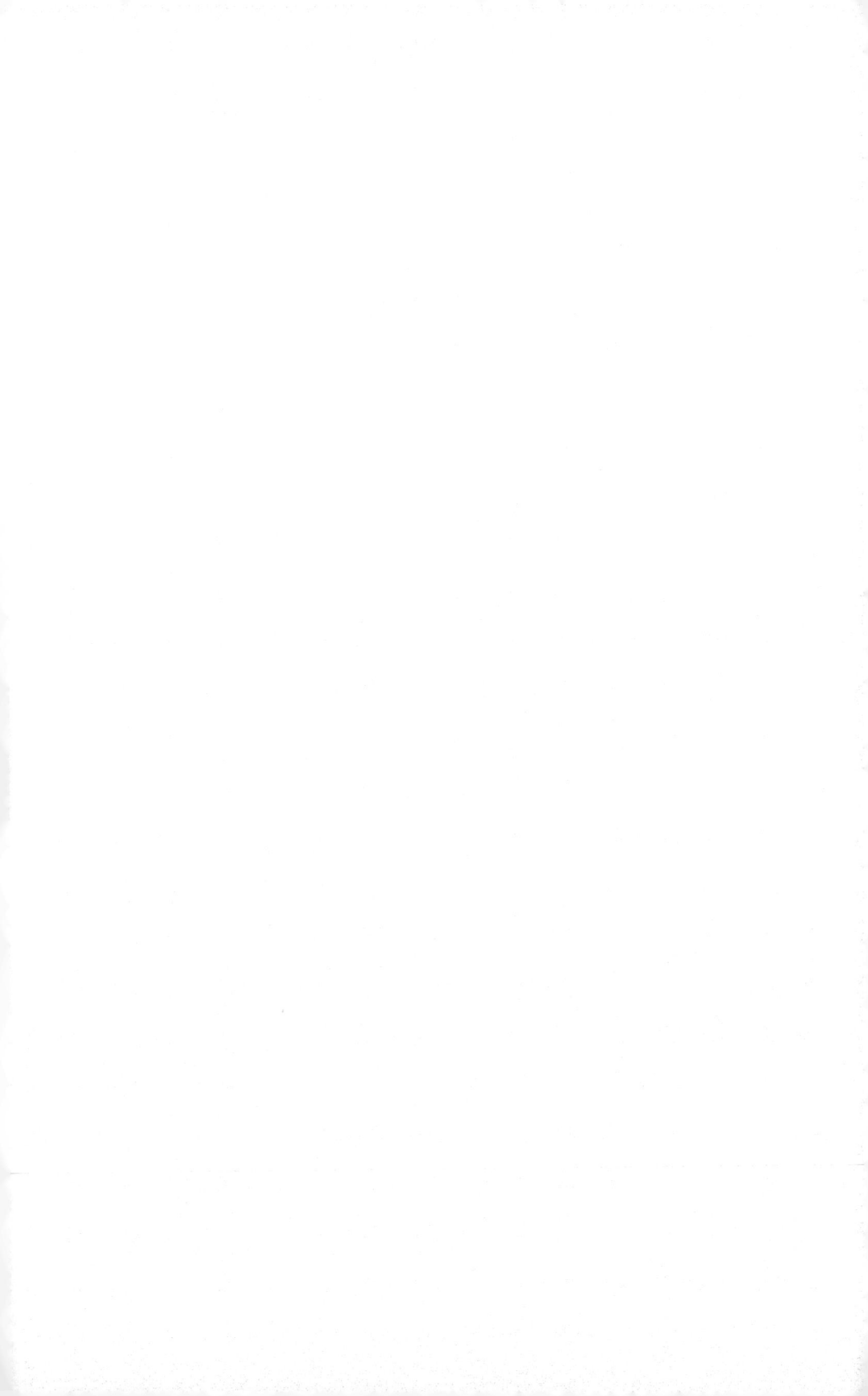

Printed in Great Britain
by Amazon